Communication in Medicine

A guide for students and physicians on interacting with
patients, colleagues, and everyone else

Kimberly J. Kinder, MD

Contents

Dedication:

This book is dedicated to my wonderful husband Jesse. Without him, I could not have made it through medical school and residency to be where I am now.

Acknowledgements:

I wish to thank all of the people who taught me how to communicate effectively. I also appreciate the examples of ineffective communication, but will not name those individuals. The person who has given me the most inspiration for writing this book (although he doesn't know it) is Dr. Joseph Carter. He helped me when I was struggling with communication skills and is the ultimate example of the type of doctor I would want to have as a patient and colleague. Dr. Maroun Semaan was probably the most patient surgeon I have ever seen in trying to walk a junior resident through a procedure. He effectively explained how to do something and why we were doing it. Dr. Pierre Lavertu always made time to answer the cancer patient's "just one more question."

Introduction

About the book:

I wish this book had been around when I was going through medical school and residency. I am the first physician in my family, so although I spoke with people in the medical field before I started my medical training, I had no idea what I was getting myself into. Memorizing the Kreb's cycle and the 20 muscles in the forearm, changing to another rotation in medical school as soon as you start to get the hang of the previous one, and surviving sleepless hours on call were all challenges. However, I think what might have actually challenged me most was learning how to communicate effectively with everyone I encountered. This is something I'm still working on, but I think I have made a lot of progress. I want to share all of the things I have learned with you here. This is not intended to be a book with a lot of references or scientific data, so you will not be able to list it as "evidence-based medicine." The "evidence," though, is that I am a practicing physician who hears positive feedback from my patients, colleagues, and mentors. I still get some negative feedback, but I am working on that.

This book is written for individuals at many different training levels — medical students, residents, and fully-licensed practicing physicians. I am drawing on experiences from all of those levels. Some of the things I have learned most recently would have been great to know before I ever saw a patient in medical school. At the same time, it is never too late to learn these skills.

I have talked about concepts in general and also provided specific examples. These include situations throughout medical school, residency, and my current practice. I have changed names and details whenever needed for confidentiality.

About me:

I grew up in a small town in Michigan. My mom was a school psychologist and my dad worked in research and development for the infant formula division of a pharmaceutical company. I have one younger sister. Education was always stressed in my family, so I knew I was going to college when I was done with high school. I had a strong interest in science from an early age, so I just figured I was going to be a doctor.

I did my undergraduate studies at a small liberal arts school in Indiana called DePauw University. I majored in East Asian Studies and spent my junior year in Japan. I minored in biology, knowing all along that I planned to go to medical school. The time in Japan was great, though. Anyone who has the opportunity to spend time abroad should definitely do it as it gives you an appreciation of the positive AND negative aspects of American society by learning firsthand about another culture. The other great thing about college was that I met my husband there. He was planning to go to graduate school for physics and was two years ahead of me. He looked all around the country and decided to go to the University of Pennsylvania in Philadelphia since there were four medical schools in the city. We figured this would give me the best chance of getting into a school in the same city.

I finished my undergraduate degree and moved to Philadelphia. I spent a year doing basic science research at a biology laboratory at Thomas Jefferson University (which in large part has prompted the chapter on working with researchers). The next summer, I married Jesse and started medical school at Penn. Med school was challenging — academically at first and physically later. Penn had a course called "Doctoring" which went through all four years and focused on the social side of medicine — the doctor-patient relationship, medical ethics, and teamwork. I'm sure that some of the things I learned in that course have made their way into this book, but time in a classroom could not really prepare me for the events out in the trenches.

I found in medical school that I really enjoyed surgery, and decided to specialize in ENT (ear, nose, and throat surgery, AKA otolaryngology, AKA otorhinolaryngology). I think it is probably the most poorly-named specialty, but other than that, it is pretty good. I get to see patients in the clinic and care for them medically as well as do a wide variety of surgical procedures. I matched at University Hospitals — Case Medical Center in Cleveland, Ohio. My intern year was shared with general surgery and ENT, so I got to rotate through general surgery, transplant surgery, vascular surgery, the surgical ICU, anesthesia, oral surgery, pediatric surgery, neurosurgery, trauma surgery, and ENT. I started in the ICU and was soon in over my head. When being asked about pressor choice and dosage, I sure was grateful that the ICU nurse was there to help me.

There was a lot to learn academically in residency, but the hardest thing for me at that time was the sleep deprivation. I made sure to comply with the 80-hour work week restriction, but those 80 hours did not include the time I had to spend at home preparing for the next day's cases, general studying, and presentations. I think I was sort of a zombie and didn't really realize it until I had a week of vacation and could feel again what it was like not to be physically, mentally, and emotionally exhausted. In this limited functional capacity, I was supposed to learn how to be a good doctor. How can you be pleasant and caring to those around you when you can't even keep your eyes open standing at a surgical table? I had some challenges in this regard that I will describe later. I did get through it, though, and finished the 5-year residency on schedule.

My husband and I have always enjoyed the West. So when we were trying to figure out where to go after I finished residency, we looked at a lot of western cities. We decided on Albuquerque, NM for multiple reasons: strong need for ENTs, excellent physics research opportunities, over 300 days of sun per year, and lots of outdoor activities nearby. I am a hospital-employed physician and have 3 ENT partners. I have more free time now than I ever had in medical school or residency and enjoy my current work-life balance. Jesse and I do not have any children and are not sure if we will, but we are happy where we are at this point. That brings you up to speed on me, so now on to the rest of the book.

SECTION ONE: Communication with Patients

Chapter 1: Starting the doctor-patient relationship

I remember the jitters I felt in medical school the first time I had to see a patient. Now I see 20 or more per day in my outpatient clinic. The nervousness has gone away as I have gained confidence in my skills, but you always want to start a relationship with a new patient properly. Here are my keys:

1. Introduce yourself.

It sounds simple, but we sometimes forget. When I go into an exam room, I shake the patient's hand and say my first and last name. I do not introduce myself as "Dr. Kinder" since some patients seem put off by that, but then I do occasionally have patients that ask later on, "Are you my doctor?" I don't wear a white coat in clinic, either, so this can add to the confusion.

In my experience, the further along we get in our practice, the less we cling to formalities. This applies to both the white coat and how we have patients address us. I always wore my white coat as a medical student. In residency, it depended on the situation. I was so happy in residency that I was finally a doctor that I always introduced myself as "Dr. Kinder." Now it doesn't matter so much. What you go by depends on your practice environment and personal preference.

The patients should have some idea how to address you, but the more important thing is that they know your role. In medical school, you should tell the patient you are a medical student and that you are working with Dr. X or are on the Y team (pulmonary, surgery, etc.). Then the patient has some sense of how to frame the interaction with you. Many patients have a hard time understanding how compartmentalized medicine has become, but you can at least try to help them understand where you fit in.

2. Maintain positive body language.

You may be the most brilliant physician in the world, but if you never make eye contact with the patient, he probably won't listen to what you say. It's often said that you only have one chance to make a first impression, and this is very true in medicine. Whether you are meeting a patient in the hospital, emergency room, or clinic, the patient's impression of you is largely framed by that first encounter. Make eye contact and appear interested in what the patient is saying. The patient may not know what information is relevant (and you may not know until later, either). If you are using a computer/electronic medical record (EMR) at the same time, make sure you take time to look at the patient either while typing or in between sentences. Try to get on the same eye level with the patient if possible. If you are as exhausted as I was during residency, you will enjoy the chance to sit down, as well. Try not to cross your arms. Position yourself at an appropriate distance from the patient. Don't be so close that the patient feels intimidated, but don't be so far that it seems you are not interested.

3. Try not to interrupt.

After you have introduced yourself, give the patient some time to tell you what she thinks is important about why she is seeing you. If you do not have any information ahead of time, you may ask, "What brings you here today?" If I see someone is referred by a colleague for a specific issue, I may direct the conversation somewhat by saying, "I see Dr. Callahan sent you here for recurrent ear infections. Can you please tell me about that?" Many physicians are very impatient and we find ourselves interrupting patients before they can even complete a sentence. Most patients will only talk for 1-2 minutes at most before they stop. If you do not believe me, time it the next time you are in a clinic. If you do have a patient that keeps going and you know you are not getting the information you need, then it may be appropriate to interrupt. The majority of the time, it is really the physician's impatience at trying to "get to the point" rather than the patient "talking too long."

4. Try not to seem rushed.

We all know that there are a lot of time pressures in medicine. One of the nice things about being a medical student is that you often have the least time pressure. On my internal medicine rotation, I was assigned 1-2 patients at a time, so I had all day to focus on them. I've heard from a number of patients over the years that they enjoy having medical students on their team since the medical students actually spend time listening to them.

The trick as you move on to having a higher patient census is learning how to spend fewer minutes per patient while still making them feel heard. Some of this relates to making eye contact and maintaining positive body language. Additionally, make sure that you are not constantly looking at your watch or tapping your foot. In situations where you are very busy, you may have to tell the patient that you only have 10 minutes to talk before you have to go to surgery. In true emergencies, you may have very little time for conversation, but you then need to go back to the patient once the emergency is over and make sure that his needs have been addressed. If you have only 15-20 minutes for a clinic visit, you may have to tell the patient that you cannot address all of her concerns today, but you are happy to schedule a follow up visit to talk about additional issues.

5. Get to know patients if you can.

This is really "continuing" the doctor-patient relationship rather than starting it, but a lot of this is initiated when you first meet a patient. Outside of certain situations in medical school, we usually do not have endless hours to spend with an individual patient. However, both you and the patient will enjoy the relationship more if you know a little about Mrs. Jones as a person and not just "the diabetic lady with end-stage renal disease." I do have a surgeon mentality, so I generally enjoyed doing things rather than talking about things in medical school. Because of this, I think I may have lost some opportunities to really get to know patients.

Knowing more about the patient as a person is sometimes critical to the care you are providing. For example, if your patient has dementia and you need to address end-of-life care, you need to know the family dynamics and who is making decisions. A patient may not take a medication you prescribe because he just lost his job and can't pay for it, not because he is being "non-compliant." I've had many patients come to me because they had mild sore throats and were worried they had cancer because their friends had died after having similar symptoms.

In addition, knowing patients helps you remember them and enjoy your job. Even though I am a specialist, I have some patients that follow up with me on a regular basis. I see a lot of patients with ear infections, but remembering that Mr. Martinez was the retired history professor who moved here from Texas helps him stand out. I look forward to hearing about the 80th birthday party, recent cruise, or updates on the kids. I've spoken with a number of primary care doctors who really enjoy this aspect of medicine, but I know it can get overwhelming at times. Patients usually like it when you are interested in them as people, too. You clearly need to get through certain medical information each time you have an encounter with a patient, but we would be scientists instead of physicians if we didn't have at least some interest in caring for people.

Chapter 2: Explain things — truthfully!

Each person is an expert in something. Soon after we moved to New Mexico, we had problems with our washing machine sending water all over the floor. I happened to be home when the repairman came. I watched what he was doing and talked to him as he fixed it. He explained what he was doing, so if the same thing happened again, I think I would be able to fix it. He clearly knew much more than I do about washing machines, but he was able to teach me what I needed to know. We need to do the same thing for our patients. We do not expect them to spend 25+ years of their lives in training to be able to remove a gallbladder, but we need to clearly explain the risks, benefits, and recovery process.

1. Explanations in general

I often end up going over my 15-20 minute scheduled visit time in the clinic because I find myself explaining a lot of things to patients. I know my explanations need to get more concise, but I would definitely prefer that a patient hears too much rather than not enough. You do have to assess the patient's level of interest and background knowledge before you start your explanation to make sure you maximize its effect. Do not make the mistake of being too technical. Even if your patient is a medical professional, she might not know all of your specialty-specific terminology. As an ENT, I don't remember off the top of my head which tarsal bone is which even though I had to learn about them in medical school.

I see several benefits to explaining things. First, if patients understand what is going on, they are more likely to feel like you helped them even if you could not make their problem go away. Second, they are more likely to adhere to treatments you prescribe if they know why you are suggesting them. Third, you are less likely to be sued (or at least found guilty) if you have adequately explained a procedure. Finally, I enjoy being able to teach others. To undertake the life-long learning needed to be a physician, I hope we all at least have some interest in sharing some of that information we acquired!

With any explanation, the most important thing is to be truthful. If you do not know something, do not make it up. It is much better to admit that you do not know than to lie. If it is something you can look up and get back to the patient, great. If it is something that the medical community as a whole does not know or understand, let the patient know that. It is constantly humbling to me how much we still need to learn about the human body.

2. Explain the diagnosis.

Some patients come in already knowing what is wrong, but many do not. I feel that part of my job as a physician is to tell the patient what is happening (or at least what I think is happening). It is often helpful to have diagrams or models when explaining anatomic issues since it can be hard for patients to visualize what is going on under the skin. I see in my practice that many patients do not differentiate between the nose itself and the sinuses. I often show them on illustrated wall charts where the sinuses are located, the structures inside the nose, and how each of these is related to the symptoms they experience.

Sometimes explanations can be simple, like telling a patient he has a broken leg. Other things can be complex, like explaining diabetic ketoacidosis to the family member of an obtunded patient. Discussing a diagnosis can become more complex, though, depending on how much detail you provide on anatomy, physiology, and pathophysiology. The level of detail should be tailored to the patient's background, interest, and questions. There are also time limits to consider in many situations.

3. Explain the treatment.

After the patient knows what's wrong, you need to explain the next step(s). This may involve further testing. If you are ordering any kind of test, you should tell the patient why. This may be as simple as saying, "We are ordering a CT scan with contrast to see what this lump is in your neck. We also need to order a blood test to make sure your kidneys are OK before we give you the IV dye for the CT." This takes about 10 seconds to say, but makes the process much clearer to the patient than just giving him an order slip.

The rationale behind a medication or treatment needs to be discussed, as well. For example, "I am prescribing Lisinopril because it should both lower your blood pressure and help protect your kidneys from damage associated with high blood pressure." In a patient with acute appendicitis, you may say, "I recommend we take your appendix out today so it does not rupture and cause a more serious infection." Some of these things seem very basic to us after our training, but someone without the same training may not make some of these connections automatically.

If tests or treatment are invasive or painful, you need to tell the patient. None of us like pain, but it is especially bad if no one warns us. In ENT residency, we practiced the flexible fiberoptic nasal exam on each other to learn how to do it. Whenever I am doing this procedure for a patient, I tell her that I have had it done to myself and what to expect. Patients like to know if you have been through something and can empathize with them.

You should explain as much as you can about the course of testing and treatment. You may have to tell the patient that you can not say much until you get the results of certain tests, but you need to share that information once it is available. Patients need to know how long you are planning to put them on a medication (a couple weeks vs indefinitely), how long a treatment will take (a single dose of radioactive iodine for thyroid cancer vs 5-7 weeks of daily radiation treatments for a throat cancer), and suspected or potential side effects of a treatment.

If you are not the person making the ultimate decision about a test or treatment, you should not give the patient false information. For example, I see a number of pediatric patients in my office who have problems with their tonsils. The parents will sometimes tell me that the pediatrician said the child needed her tonsils out. Guidelines for tonsillectomy are constantly changing, so we do a lot fewer tonsillectomies now than at other times in history. It is extra work for me to explain why the child does NOT actually need her tonsils out than if the pediatrician had said to the parent, "Go see Dr. Kinder to see if she thinks you need tonsil surgery." When I refer to another specialist, I will sometimes mention treatments that they MIGHT prescribe, but I never try to tell a patient what another doctor SHOULD do.

4. Explain procedures — "Informed Consent"

This section is probably most important to surgeons and physicians who do office- or hospital-based procedures, but every physician needs to know about it. The most important part of explaining a procedure is to make sure you know what you are talking about. When I was in residency, it was often the job of the intern or the junior resident to obtain the procedural consent from the patient in the pre-op area. The attending surgeon should have already discussed that procedure with the patient in the office, but if the patient had questions that I could not answer, I should not have been getting the consent. I made sure as a senior resident to caution my junior residents about this so we could make sure we were giving the patients the correct information.

We often think the main reason we explain procedures is so we can get a patient to provide "Informed Consent." "Informed Consent" is NOT the patient's signature on a document detailing the risks of surgery. It is the PROCESS you go through with the patient to make sure you both know what you are doing and why you are doing it. Even though a patient signed the form, he can still say he did not give "Informed Consent." It is your obligation to try to make sure you have really informed the patient before doing anything invasive.

If you are not the one doing the procedure, do not provide details that may be incorrect. This applies most to medical students and residents, but can also apply in referring patients to other providers. If you don't know something, it is always better to admit that than to make something up. You may have to ask the person who is actually doing the procedure so you can provide the correct information to the patient. For example, I sometimes refer patients to general surgeons for consideration of acid reflux surgery. If the patients ask me any details, I tell them that it is usually done laparoscopically (since that is the trend at my institution), but that the general surgeon would be able to tell them a lot more.

Make sure that you tell the patient about any expected side effects of a procedure as well as possible risks. For example, if you are doing a total thyroid-ectomy, you should tell the patient she will have to take thyroid replacement medication for the rest of her life. This is an expected side effect of the surgery. You also need to tell her about the possible risks of hoarseness, breathing issues, and low calcium. These are known potential complications, but only happen in a small percentage of patients. You should be prepared with the next steps should any of these complications occur (i.e. calcium supplementation, tracheostomy) but can choose whether or not to discuss these with the patient. Your risk discussion for any procedure should include both common complications and rare but serious complications.

Chapter 3: Ensure understanding

After you have explained the diagnosis, treatment, and procedure, you need to make sure patients have actually understood these things. I have had encounters where I thought I did a great job explaining the reason for a medication to a patient, only to see him again in a month to learn he never took the medicine. Some of the information below overlaps with things I have discussed earlier, but we know that repetition aids retention.

1. Avoid technical terms (when possible).

I may know what a proton pump inhibitor is, but my patient may not. It makes much more sense to most patients to tell them that omeprazole stops the acid from actually being formed rather than just blocking the acid like ranitidine. I will often mention technical terms to patients but always try to explain them in basic terms, as well. For example, I will tell a patient that he will see "dysphagia" as the office visit diagnosis, which means that we talked about his problems swallowing. Most procedures and diagnoses involve technical terminology so we cannot totally avoid these things, but we need to make sure we explain any terms we use.

2. Write things down.

In many aspects of our lives, we write things down so we can remember. I make a grocery list before I go to the store so I do not forget the tomato sauce I need for a recipe. We take notes during a lecture or while reading a textbook so we can recall the important points later on. Patients often will not remember everything we say. In clinic, I have had patients tell me, "I wish I had a tape recorder so I could keep all of this information."

I don't actually record myself, but I have a lot of patient information handouts that I provide so the patients have something in writing. This includes disease-specific information (e.g. GERD and Meniere's disease handouts), medication administration instructions (PPIs and Afrin), and procedural pamphlets ("What to Expect with Tonsillectomy"). Many EMR systems come with some of these handouts built in and also give you the ability to build your own. You can direct patients to reliable on-line resources, many of which have patient information sections. Each patient at my clinic is also provided with a printed "After Visit Summary" which lists the diagnosis for the visit, any medication changes, follow up instructions, the physician name, and the phone number for any questions or concerns. This is a common feature available in most EMR systems and is actually being required more and more for government reimbursement under the "meaningful use" umbrella.

3. Ask if the patient has any questions.

When I am explaining a procedure, I like to get through my explanation as much as possible without interruptions. If patients ask questions during this time, I usually ask them to let me explain as I will answer many of their questions along the way. This way I try to make sure I do not forget anything, either. When I am done, though, I always ask if the patient has any questions or concerns. I ask the same thing at the end of every office visit, seeing a patient in the hospital, or giving a post-op update to a family member. This is a very important piece of each patient interaction since you really have no idea what the patient has retained or if you have even addressed the patient's concern if you do not give him a chance to ask questions.

Some patients fail to grasp the uncertainty we often have in medicine. Their questions sometimes reveal this. We usually try to tell patients what we EXPECT or HOPE will happen after an intervention, but many patients assume that something we say in this situation definitely WILL happen. When I do a septoplasty, I tell the patient it will not cure his sleep apnea, but that it generally will make the CPAP easier to use and we might be able to lower his airway pressure.

4. Repetition

Repetition is important (as you can see). If something is very important, it often helps to repeat it. This is especially true if you are providing the patient a lot of information at once. Repetition can be in the form of verbally saying something twice at the same visit, reinforcing concepts over subsequent visits, or written instructions. It can also be helpful to have patients tell you what you just said to make sure they are understanding it properly.

Chapter 4: The patient and the family

The patient sometimes presents to you as an individual, but many patients have families that you need to treat, as well. We have to remember that the patient always comes first, but we usually cannot (and should not) exclude the families.

1. Minor patients

Except in certain situations (i.e. emancipated minor, STD treatment, true medical emergencies), a minor needs to have a parent or legal guardian present. The exclusions vary from state-to-state, so make sure you are aware of your state's laws. The parent or legal guardian usually needs to be physically present for you to be allowed to interview or examine a minor patient. If the adult with the minor is not the biological parent, you need to have paperwork on file that shows the adult is allowed to make decisions for that minor.

In addition to making sure you are legally compliant as above, you want to include the family of a minor patient since the patient often needs the help of the family to follow through with treatment. This is obvious in young children, but even teens often have limited understanding since teenage brains are not wired the same as adult brains. Minors often need parents to transport them to medical facilities, administer treatments, and help them understand why something is being done.

Parents usually know their children much better than you do, so you need to listen to what parents say.

This does not mean you always have to do what they tell you, but you need to at least hear their concerns. A father may tell you that his daughter seems to be having a harder time paying attention, which may make you suspect pediatric sleep apnea. A lot of children have large tonsils, but only a limited subset actually needs tonsillectomy. If the child is symptomatic, she may be one who would benefit from surgery. On the other hand, a mother may tell you she thinks her son has an ear infection since he is fussy and pulling at his ear. If you see that the ear is clear and you think this issue is due to teething, you do not have to prescribe the antibiotics she wants. Parents may not always be medical experts, but most of them DO know their children at least to some extent.

You need to explain things both to the parents and the patient as much as possible. When preparing for a tonsillectomy in a 4-year-old, I will tell the parents about the risks and benefits. I also tell the child directly that it will be very important for her to drink lots of juice and water after the surgery even if it hurts. There is a wide range of maturity levels in children, so I try to include in the discussion any child that seems to be paying attention (which seems to start anywhere from age 3 to 10).

In minor patients that are old enough to understand things, you need to get "assent" from the patient and "consent" from the parent when doing any procedure. The age for this varies, so you generally have to use your judgement. This is especially important when there is not a true right or wrong answer about what to do and when the procedure requires some cooperation on the part of the patient. I see a lot of teenagers with sports-related nasal bone fractures in my office. The parent, patient, and I have to make the decision together whether or not to do surgery to try to improve the nasal alignment. If the 16-year-old basketball player is not bothered by the fact that his nose is a little crooked and he just wants to keep playing basketball (rather than protecting the nose during the healing period), it does not make a lot of sense to do a surgery. The parent has to agree with this, of course, but we need to all try to get on the same page.

2. The "Impaired" patient

We think of most adults as being in charge of their own medical care, but this is not always true. Patients may be temporarily or permanently unable to make decisions for themselves. This can be an obtunded patient after a motorcycle crash, a hospitalized patient with delirium, a patient with mental retardation, or an elderly patient with severe Alzheimer's disease. If there is documentation that directs our care (Healthcare Power of Attorney, Living Will, etc.), we need to follow what is written on the document. We are often caught in situations where documentation is not available, though. In these situations, we need to first determine whether or not the patient is actually able to make his own decisions. This can be easy or difficult. If there is any question, you can request a competency assessment (usually from the psychiatry or medicine department) or help from the legal department at your hospital.

If a patient is not able to make his own decisions, we need to determine who should be doing this. If there are multiple family members and they all agree with each other, you listen to the family. In situations where there is disagreement among family members, your hospital can give you a list in rank order (i.e. spouse, then adult children, then parents, then siblings). As the primary medical professional caring for a patient in this situation, do not be afraid to ask for help from the ethics or legal departments of your facility if you have any concerns.

We often get overwhelmed when there are many family members involved. We want to try to address everyone's needs and concerns, but we have to be reasonable. It saves you a lot of time and frustration to set expectations at the beginning of caring for these patients, especially in the inpatient setting. It can often be helpful to identify 1 or 2 contact people so you do not have to explain things over and over to 20 different family members. You can also set up times for family meetings to give updates on the overall plan of care.

3. Cancer patients

Patients with many different types of cancer need a lot of support, both from inside and outside of the medical system. In my experience, cancer patients who have a strong support network of family or friends tend to do better than those who do not. We cannot generally change a patient's social network, but we need to include these people in the patient's care.

When a patient hears a diagnosis of cancer, she often does not hear much else of what you say at that time. If you have not yet experienced this, you will. In talking to cancer patients, you often need to repeat things multiple times and explain things in multiple ways. Each time, a little bit more information seems to sink in. The families can sometimes help with this, but other families have a harder time understanding things than the patient. I try to encourage cancer patients to have friends or family come with them to office visits so we can all discuss things together.

Cancer patients often need their family members to take them to radiation and chemotherapy sessions. There are also office visits with primary care physicians, medical oncologists, radiation oncologists, and sometimes surgeons. Patients may require care from nutritionists or physical, occupational, or speech therapists. Patients sometimes talk about a "chemo fog," so you need to make sure a responsible adult is able to care for these patients and comprehend instructions.

Families are often financially, physically, and emotionally challenged when a member of the family is diagnosed with cancer. Many oncology departments and hospital systems have services specifically designed to help with these challenges. The "Cancer Nurse Navigator" is becoming a popular role to help patients and families navigate the system. Although only one person is diagnosed with cancer, it usually affects the entire family.

4. Families in general

Many patients who are not in the specific situations listed above also want their families involved with their care. Families are often interested in knowing what is wrong with their loved ones. A patient may depend on her family to help her get through an illness or recover from a surgery. Some patients like to involve their spouses or other family members in their medical decisions, even if they are able to make a decision on their own. We need to respect this and try to keep everyone informed.

Families can become your allies, as well. A family member can often help remember details — "Don't forget to tell the doctor about your stroke" — or provide more accurate information — "You've been having a hard time breathing for a few years, not just a couple months." Getting families involved can help a patient do a better job adhering to your recommendations. I have a number of elderly patients that come with their adult children to the office. The adult children are oftentimes the ones keeping track of the list of medications and getting the parents to the visits. I make sure to talk to both the patient and the family to make sure the necessary information is transmitted.

Chapter 5: Cultural and language differences

We live in a very diverse country, so we need to know how to communicate with people who come from different backgrounds. This section is not intended to make you an expert in various cultural norms, but to try to make you aware of some general "do's" and "don'ts."

1. Cultural diversity

This shows up in a variety of ways. When I was in residency, I generally shook hands with my patients when introducing myself. I went to shake the hand of the father of my 5-year-old patient, and he would not shake my hand. I did not push the situation, but I did not understand. I later learned from a colleague that my patient and his father were Hassidic Jews and he considered it improper to touch me since I was a female. There is no way we can possibly learn all of the nuances for the many cultures we come in contact with, but we need to respect these differences.

The first thing I would advise is this: Try not to be offended. Females in certain cultures only want to be examined by other females. We can try to accommodate this when possible, but it is not always an option. The patient then has a choice if she wants to be treated or not. People from certain cultures may not respect me because I am a woman who has a job and I do not keep my hair and body covered. I do not have to change who I am, but I can still be professional in my work interactions.

Second, try not to be offensive. Many cultures have different norms in communication. You will not know all these norms, but you do not want to push people into something with which they are uncomfortable. If you pick up on signals, try to listen to them. You will probably at some point unintentionally offend someone, but at least try to be careful. If you have a large population of a certain cultural group in your geographic area, try to learn some of the differences so you are prepared for these encounters.

One of the differences we see in many cultures is patient-centered versus family-centered decision making. We tend to be very individualistic in America. In other societies, though, the family will want to make the decisions for the patient. I had a Chinese family tell me that I could not tell my 80-year-old patient that he had cancer. They did not want him to know, and they wanted to make the treatment choices. This is the opposite of what we are taught when learning about the doctor-patient relationship in our training. I expressed to the family my concerns and we eventually got to tell the patient together about his diagnosis, but it was a challenging situation. I generally feel that the patient has the right to know about his own medical situation due to the way I was raised and trained. If you are having problems with cultural differences like this, you can try first to work with the family and then involve the ethics or legal departments if needed.

We often think of "cultural sensitivity" as relevant to people from other countries or religious traditions, but it can also apply to someone who grew up in a different setting from you. We cannot assume that a person has the same cultural norms just because he grew up in the same city. Based on his upbringing, an individual may have a style of speech or dress you find offensive or incomprehensible, or a confrontational attitude toward you as a person or health care provider. We need to make sure that we acknowledge these issues so we can effectively help our patients. We may need to ask more follow up questions in interviewing. For example, if I ask how long a patient has had a cough and she says, "A minute," I need to clarify if that means a couple of weeks, months, or years. When a patient tells me that he "rarely" drinks alcohol, further questioning has revealed that to mean anything from several drinks per day to several drinks per year. Non-specific words mean different things to different people, so make sure you clarify.

2. Foreign languages

We will all encounter patients that do not speak our language. This includes both foreign travelers and residents who have not learned English. Some of my colleagues in New Mexico speak Spanish as well as English, but I do not. If you want to learn a second language, that is great. However, it is likely that we will all have to use interpreters at some point.

A true interpreter is someone who fluently speaks both languages and can transmit the nuances of one language appropriately into another. An interpreter should tell the patient exactly what you said, changing only certain words or thoughts that do not translate into the other language. Whenever the patient says something, the interpreter should translate it directly to you rather than trying to answer the question on her own. This is what formally trained interpreters will do, whether they are present in person, on a video screen, or on a telephone.

In some settings, we do not have true interpreters, but just people who can speak both languages. In my clinic, many of the medical assistants speak Spanish and English. When a Spanish-speaking patient presents for an office visit, a medical assistant may come into the room with me and "interpret." However, I notice that they sometimes try to answer questions on their own, so I may not know what is being said for a couple minutes. This still works in most situations, but can be somewhat frustrating as I don't always know what advice is being given.

The final type of interpretation we frequently see is by family members. In many families that live in New Mexico, at least one family member has learned English. If this person comes to the visit, he often interprets for the patient. When I see this happening, I always ask the patient if she is comfortable having the family member interpret or if she wants us to bring another person in. I think some information from the patient gets lost when the family member is translating, because the family member will often provide the history for the patient and only actually ask the patient my questions when not sure of an answer.

Clearly, the most important thing is to be able to communicate with the patient. This includes getting the information you need to do your job and providing the patient with the information he needs to get better. This can often be accomplished with any of the above interpreting schemes. You also want to try to connect with the patient on a personal level. Although it is generally agreed that a fully-trained interpreter does the best job transmitting all of the information, some patients and families will be offended if you do not let the family member interpret. Therefore, if it seems like the family member is generally getting the big picture across, I usually let him interpret. However, when it comes to more legal issues, such as consent for a procedure, I make sure I have a fully trained interpreter to help with those details. If the patient or family is upset that I am bringing another person in, I will usually say something like, "I want to make sure we get all of the important information to everyone, which is sometimes hard with some of the technical words we need to use."

It is helpful to know how to appropriately use an interpreter, as well. You should look at the patient when you are talking, even though she may not understand what you are saying. You still want to use the techniques we talked about in establishing the doctor-patient relationship. Make sure you speak clearly and in short enough sentences or phrases so the interpreter does not have to remember a long explanation all at once. These visits are going to take longer, so try not to get frustrated. If you are using a video translation service, it is most important that the patient can see the screen since the sound can sometimes be sub-optimal. The patient may not be trained in speaking clearly and concisely, so it is most important that she and the interpreter can see each other if possible. Do not forget to ask if the patient has any questions, just like you would with any other patient.

Chapter 6: The difficult patient

We would love it if all of our patients provided concise and accurate histories, followed our advice, and got better. This is not the world of medicine, though. You will have at least one of these issues with many patients, but hopefully will have a limited number of truly "difficult" patients. There are a number of different things that can make a patient "difficult." We will discuss several below.

1. The talker

Some people love to talk. When you are making morning rounds or trying to get through 15-minute clinic slots, this can bring you to a grinding halt. You need to be armed with skills to make sure you get the information you need, address the patient's concerns, and do not get stuck spending your entire day with one patient.

In some situations, it may be OK just to let the person talk. If you are a primary care physician and are seeing a stable patient for annual medication refills, as long as the patient says he is doing fine with his current regime, you may be able to let him spend the office visit talking about whatever he desires. You can sometimes check or order labs on the computer while he is talking. I find that I can listen and type at the same time fairly effectively.

If you have a lot of questions that you have to get through and the patient really does not stop talking, you may have to interrupt. Like I said earlier, most patients will not talk for more than a few minutes when you give them free reign at the beginning, so you need to give your "talker" this time, too. If the patient just keeps going, you can say, "I see Dr. Mitchell sent you here to talk about your acid reflux. When did that start?" Rather than asking open-ended questions, you may need to ask very specific questions. I find that many of my "talkers" will answer a question like this at the beginning, even though they may then launch into a seemingly long explanation.

If the patient keeps discussing things that are seemingly off-topic, you can often be looking back and forth between the patient and the chart to find some of the information you need. Mention in your note where you are getting information if it is not coming from the patient. You may also need to directly tell the patient that you only have 15 minutes together and you need to get through certain things. Alternatively, you may be able to say, "We only have 15 minutes, but you can talk about what you think is most important with me during that time." This is usually feasible in a clinic environment, but you may have to be more focused in the hospital setting.

2. The "poor historian"

Sometimes it can be really hard to get a history from a patient. This can be because they are a "talker," or they may not talk enough. Again, when patients are not freely volunteering the information you desire, it is best to ask simple, direct questions. "Where do you feel the pain? Is it worse when you lie down?" Some patients contradict themselves. For example, a patient told me she had not tried any medications for her allergies, but I saw Claritin on her medication list. She then said, "Oh, I tried that for a month." This can be incredibly frustrating. I often have to ask for clarification in these situations to find out which information is correct. I will usually mention some of the contradictions in my note to remind myself in case I have to go back and look at things.

Some patients appear quite uninformed about their medical histories. They may not remember details of surgeries, which medications they take, and what kind of doctors they see. It is very helpful in these situations to have an EMR that carries this information forward. I will also ask patients if they have a family member or primary doctor who can help me obtain this information if needed. I usually ask a patient if he has any medical problems. If he says, "no," I will list specific things that are common or may be important in my caring for him (i.e. diabetes, hypertension, asthma). With surgeries, you can look for scars during your physical exam and ask where they came from. If you work hard at it, you can often get a fair amount of information even from the "poor historian."

We should not label a patient a "poor historian" if we are just not doing a good job obtaining the information. I feel like it is often more helpful to write something like, "patient jumps from topic to topic," "patient unsure which medications he takes," or "patient provides contradictory information about symptoms," rather than just writing, "poor historian." If you know why the patient is having a hard time, you should document this, as well. For example, if you are trying to examine a patient who recently had head trauma, this could be why an otherwise lucid person cannot give you the information you want. A patient may have just received pain medication in the hospital, be unable to speak well after a stroke, or have dementia.

3. The demanding patient

A patient may come to you with a diagnosis and treatment already in mind. As a physician or physician-in-training, it is your job to try to determine if the diagnosis and treatment are correct. I just had a patient that complained of pressure in his ears and decided he had an infection. He actually got his primary care doctor to prescribe him some topical antibiotic ear drops over the phone without examining him, but wanted me to give him different ones since the first were too expensive. I looked in his ears and saw no sign of infection, so told him I would not prescribe or recommend antibiotics. He was not happy, but we continued to talk and I explained the correct treatment for what I diagnosed as his problem.

Saying "no" to a patient is especially difficult when you are just starting your training. We want to try to get along with patients, but our primary goal is really to provide appropriate medical care. In my "doctoring" class in medical school, we had a standardized patient who portrayed a mother who wanted antibiotics for her child who had a viral illness. One of my classmates was playing the physician, and he was clearly uncomfortable. The mother character was very pushy and kept raising objections when my classmate continued declining. He eventually said to her, "In my expert opinion, you should take soup." We all got a kick out of this. The student turned to us after the scenario and said, "After 18 years of school, all I've got is soup."

Even though it was funny at the time, these situations can be very frustrating. If you know you are right, you have to stick to your guns. You probably don't want to say, "In my expert opinion," but you do need to let the patient know why you disagree. You can say, "We've done research studies that show that antibiotics don't help people get better from a viral infection. We also worry that if we use antibiotics too much, they won't work anymore when we need them." Some patients will be convinced, but others will not.

You will sometimes be asked to order unnecessary or inappropriate tests by patients. I try to figure out why a patient wants a certain test. I find that this is often a situation where a patient is misinformed rather than being pushy. For example, a patient may complain of vision changes and want me to order an MRI because she saw on the internet that she might have a brain tumor. I would generally suggest that the patient see an ophthalmologist first for a thorough eye exam before proceeding to a costly and perhaps unneeded test.

Offering a second opinion can be helpful, as well, if the patient is asking for something that you do not think is right. This is usually best when the patient's request is not totally unreasonable. For example, I do not feel that most patients with mild sinus disease on a CT scan would be helped by surgery. However, some ENTs have different criteria. If a patient in this situation really wants surgery, I can offer to send him to a colleague to see what that person thinks. By doing so, I have maintained my integrity but still given the patient an option. If the patient's request is totally unreasonable, a referral is unlikely to help.

A particular class of "demanding" patients we often see are the ones we label as "drug-seekers." These patients will ask you for narcotics even when you do not see a clear indication for them. It is true that pain is subjective, but we do not want to encourage narcotic abuse. You can usually run a check through your state pharmacy board to see how many narcotic scripts have been filled by a patient and through which pharmacies and providers. I explain to these patients that I will not prescribe them narcotics because I do not see a reason on physical exam to give the medication. I will refer them to pain management if they desire. I also tell them that if they are truly in severe pain, they can go to the emergency room. I do not want to encourage overuse or abuse of the emergency room, but I do need to give the patient an option.

4. The "non-compliant" patient

We want patients to take our advice and follow our recommendations, but this does not always happen. We labeled these patients "non-compliant" when I was in medical school, but I have heard people talk more about "adherence" than "compliance" recently. Physicians cannot control what patients do, but we can try to encourage them to do what we think is medically correct.

Some of these patients will say, "You never told me XYZ." It is important to document in your notes what you discuss with the patient both to protect yourself and to help educate the patient. Again, printing this information can sometimes help so the patient has it in writing. You may want to have the patient repeat the information back to you, as well.

Some patients hear your recommendations but just don't follow them. The primary care doctor tells her morbidly obese diabetic patient to watch his sugar intake, take his insulin, and lose weight at each visit. However, he keeps gaining weight and his A1c is 10. It is often helpful to try to figure out the patient's reasons for not following your advice. The patient may not care about himself, but perhaps you can convince him to get a little healthier so he can be there for his daughter as she grows up. Maybe he has a hard time knowing which foods to eat, so you can have him see a nutritionist. Perhaps his knees hurt whenever he tries to walk, so you can suggest a water aerobics program. Then if he does make progress, you applaud his work and encourage him to continue.

I feel that some patients really don't understand the consequences of their actions. This seems especially common in diseases where patients have very few symptoms. Many patients with hypertension think it's "not a big deal" since they don't feel like anything is wrong. If we tell them they can go blind, destroy their kidneys and be on dialysis, or have a stroke and be paralyzed if they do not control their blood pressure, that may be a stronger motivation than just telling them to take some pills. It is nice if patients adhere to your advice without prodding, but scare tactics can sometimes be effective.

5. The patient you just don't like

You won't get along with all of your patients, just like you won't get along with every person you meet. It can be hard to provide good care for a patient when you can't wait to get away from her. In these situations, you often have to go above and beyond your usual level of care to make sure you are overcoming your bias. You may or may not have done anything wrong to make the relationship unpleasant, but you generally can't "fire" a patient just because you don't like her.

In residency, I had an experience like this as the chief resident on a busy head and neck cancer service. We would start our morning rounds anywhere between 5:30 and 6:00 A.M., seeing 10-20 patients during this time. We then had surgery from 7:00 A.M. until anywhere from 5:00 to 8:00 P.M., followed by another 30-60 minutes of rounding with the attending physicians. When we saw each patient in the morning, we had to examine wounds, check drains, see how the patient did overnight, and tell them the plan for the day. We also had junior residents writing notes and providing vital signs. As I went into each room, I would knock and then warn the patient to "watch his eyes" as we had to turn on a light. One morning, I did this and then told the patient I would have to move his pillow to examine his neck. I gently moved it and gently touched his neck. Later that day, he complained to the attending surgeon that I was "rude and rough." The team that was with me supported me in thinking that this was inaccurate, but I had to keep dealing with this patient. On subsequent days, I made sure to spend extra time with him on morning and evening rounds. I also instructed my junior residents to make sure they were extra attentive to any complaints he had during the day. I never ended up liking the guy, but I feel he still received excellent care from our team.

If you are ever really uncomfortable, make sure you have another person with you. In the hospital setting, you are often part of a team. If you have a challenging patient (i.e. she says different things to different providers, is non-adherent to your recom-mendations, or is verbally abusive), make sure you do not visit her alone. Escorts are often recommended for potentially sensitive situations, such as pelvic exams. If a patient makes me feel uncomfortable in the clinic, I have a medical assistant come into the room with me.

6. Dr. Robot

One Saturday morning, I was awakened at 6 A.M. by the pager. I called the answering service and it was a patient with a medication question. The patient was not in pain or bleeding — she just had noted insomnia for the past few days with steroids. Now I was also awake because of this patient. She said to me, "I didn't think you were sleeping. I just thought you were there."

Thankfully, some patients have a little common sense and courtesy and will not call the doctor's line at inconvenient times with non-emergency questions. However, some patients do not think of their doctors as fellow humans. I am not a robot. I need sleep. I have feelings. I do not have all of the answers. If you are mean to me, it makes it harder for me to be nice to you.

This book is not aimed at patients, so I know that writing this is not going to change patients' attitudes. The reason to include this is so that you as a medical professional are aware of the "Dr. Robot" perception. Most people would not call a friend or family member in the middle of the night unless there was an emergency, but some patients have no hesitation to call a doctor at any time for any reason. Certain specialties, programs, or practices are organized so there is no call and there is always "someone there," but a lot of after-hours medicine is done by physicians who are also working a regular schedule. Most patients do not know how this system works, but we can try to educate them to help them and ourselves. For example, if a patient has a surgery, the surgeon should tell her what to expect and what to watch out for. The surgeon or doctor's office can tell the patient that there is always a doctor on call to handle emergencies, and that other questions can be answered by the doctor during regular business hours.

In addition to not needing sleep, some patients think doctors do not have feelings. If a patient is treating you badly, you can sometimes stand up for yourself. Just a couple days before the phone call above, I was called into the emergency room at 11 P.M. after working a full day to take care of one of my partner's patients who was bleeding after a tonsillectomy. He made multiple snide comments, used profanity, and complained to his spouse about me causing him pain while I was using silver nitrate to try to stop the bleeding. I eventually said to him that I was there to help. If he wanted me to let him bleed, that was his choice, but I was trying to take care of the problem. He then turned around and became thankful and polite. It would not have been appropriate for me to start swearing at him, but it was reasonable to draw attention to his behavior, as I deserve to be treated with respect. This doesn't always work, but I was happy it did this time.

If patients are repeatedly rude or verbally abusive to you or your office staff, they can sometimes be "fired" from a practice. You and your staff must document the behavior. You then tell the patient about the behavior and that it will not be tolerated. If the behavior continues, you tell the patient that she can no longer be seen in your practice and then give the patient an option of another location where she can receive medical care. This can sometimes be tricky, so you will generally want to check with your office manager or legal department to make sure you are following all requirements so you cannot be accused of "abandoning" a patient.

SECTION TWO: Communication with Other Medical Professionals

Chapter 1: The basics

It would be nice if I said, "Patient Irving is doing well," it would be interpreted the same way no matter what my position. However, it really depends on my current level of training (i.e. medical student, resident, or fellow, and year within each of those levels), my specialty, and my track record in similar situations in the past. These factors are also important in the person who is receiving the information. In this section of the book, I will try to elucidate some of these relationships and nuances to teach you how to communicate effectively within the medical field. Most of us learn about the doctor-patient relationship in medical school, but I never received any of the following information in a classroom setting. I acquired it through trial and (unfortunately) a significant amount of error.

I have grouped together residents and fellows since they are in similar positions. I am also including interns with residents, as internship was just a part of my residency. I know that they are very separate in some training programs, though. I feel that interns, residents, and fellows share a lot of the same challenges, so it makes sense to talk about them together.

1. Be truthful.

We mentioned this in the patient communication section, but it applies here, as well. In a training environment, you will be asked questions to which you do not know the answer. DO NOT LIE! If you do not know something, admit that and then try to figure it out. This can be an academic question or a patient care issue. You want to seem intelligent to your colleagues, but the most important thing is making sure you are not jeopardizing your patients.

As a senior resident, I had several situations where junior residents told me that a patient had been afebrile overnight when the vitals had not been checked, or that the exam was normal when the intern had not actually seen the patient. When I trusted them and then found out later that I was given bad information, I was both angry at the situation and concerned for the patient. Thankfully, I did not have any serious complications from these instances, but some of my colleagues were not so lucky. It is definitely worse to get caught in a lie that endangers a patient than to get in trouble for forgetting or missing something that you own up to immediately.

Another part of being truthful is admitting if you do not know how to do something. If you are put in a situation where you are uncomfortable performing a procedure or explaining something to a patient, get help. Do NOT put your patient or yourself in danger by doing something that you are not comfortable with. For example, if you are an intern and your chief resident tells you to go drain an abscess, you need to ask your chief to help you if you do not know how to do it properly on your own.

2. Be aware of the situation.

If there were no hierarchy or politics in medicine, it would be a much easier field. However, these things exist and probably always will. You need to know where you fit in the hierarchy and communicate with people appropriately within that reference frame. You should not let errors happen. However, you will definitely struggle if you do not show the expected respect. For example, you may be the medical student on the ENT service who has been caring for Ms. Archer. You know she has a history of an artificial heart valve and should get pre-operative antibiotics. When you hear the surgeon doing the time-out prior to her thyroidectomy and the surgeon says no antibiotics are needed, you should speak up. However, you should do it in a polite way. You can say, "Dr. Lopez, I remember reading that Ms. Archer has an artificial heart valve. Do we need to give her antibiotics because of that?"

If you are at the other end of the hierarchy, do not abuse your "power" and treat people without respect. It will come back to haunt you. Nothing may happen at the time, but people who feel that they do not have power often go right past you to get you in trouble. I try to be open and honest with people and talk to them in person and privately if I have problems with them. Many people are not comfortable with this style of communication, though. I have been accused of being "mean" because I was honest with people, so you have to be careful in today's world if this is your style. People who feel powerless will often not speak to you, either. They will instead complain to a supervisor who can make trouble for you. This frustrates me because I have seen physicians in positions of power who ARE actually mean — throwing things in the OR, cursing at staff, and belittling residents in public.

The hierarchy of medical students → residents → fellows → attending physicians is fairly straightforward, but it becomes more challenging when you add in ancillary personnel. Nurses may take orders from you for medication administration or dressing changes, but you are not their boss. Physical therapists may work with your patients, but you do not know the details of their process. In general, you want to make as many allies as possible throughout the medical care team.

You should also try to learn about the critical departmental or hospital politics that affect your performance. I don't think many of us enjoy this aspect of our jobs, but you won't be very effective if you ignore it. Certain attending physicians may not get along with each other, so you probably shouldn't talk about liking how Dr. Bourne does a carpal tunnel release in front of Dr. Fernandez. Thankfully, most people try to be professional in the work setting, but you are not going to change some of the long-entrenched prejudices and behaviors. Try not to get caught in the middle of things. With any severe biases, your superiors in the hierarchy have probably faced the same issue, so you can often ask them. If you see an interaction that does not make sense, be alert for a possible political issue.

3. Do not make excuses.

It is natural in many situations for us to want to explain why we did not do something or why a certain thing happened. I painfully learned that people do not want to hear excuses. It does not matter how good the excuse is. If it sounds like an excuse when you say it, it will not go over well. Also, the lower you are on the hierarchy, the more true this is.

In residency, I had nights on call where I was busy taking care of patients the entire time. Sometimes I would finish my work and try to prepare for the next day's surgeries, but as soon as I would start to read, I would be interrupted by a pager or could not keep my eyes open due to fatigue — regularly getting only a few hours of sleep per night, waking up at 5:00 A.M., and then trying to study at 1:00 A.M. After one of these nights, my attending surgeon asked me an anatomy question that I did not know. I said that I did not know and had not gotten a chance to study that night since I was up taking care of patients all night. He said that I should have read about it the prior night rather than making excuses. I think I cried a little because that sometimes happens to me when I get very tired and frustrated. (Thank goodness I was just retracting in the surgery since I could barely keep my eyes open and they were blurry from crying!) I think his expectations were unrealistic, but that did not matter in the situation. I should have just said, "I don't know but I will look it up when we are done here."

As I got further along in residency, I got much better about not giving excuses. I established myself as a responsible resident, so most attendings I worked with knew what to expect from me. When Dr. Price asked if I had talked to the discharge coordinator about Mr. Keyes, I would say, "No, but I will have my junior resident do that as soon as possible." If Dr. Price asked why I had not done it yet, that was when I would explain that I was taking care of an emergency situation with another one of our patients. I earned a lot more respect this way than when I would start out with an excuse. As a general rule of thumb, do not give an excuse unless you are specifically asked for an explanation. Just make things right!

Chapter 2: Medical students

If you are reading this book, you probably are a medical student or have at least been one at some point. Medical school is challenging enough with the academic and physical exertion. To top it off, you are put at the bottom of a hierarchy you don't really understand and are judged on how well you can communicate with everyone else. I hope this book can help you survive!

1. Student to student

Medical school is competitive, but making another student look bad rarely makes you look good. No one likes the student who throws others "under the bus," and you almost never get away with it. You need to focus on learning as much as you can and performing as well as possible on clinical rotations. The only time you should be concerned with other students is if it can inspire you to work harder. You may not be the smartest student on the rotation, but hard work is usually noticed and appreciated.

Along these lines, try to help other students when you can. In my medical school, senior students were allowed to act as teaching assistants for the first year gross anatomy lab. I participated in this program, which was a great way to refresh my knowledge of anatomy and help the younger students. Teaching a topic tests your knowledge of it and is great preparation for the teaching you will do in residency and possibly in practice.

If you are finishing a rotation that another student is starting, give the oncoming student a sign out about the patients on the service and some of the expectations. If you picked up on any strange politics, pass this on, too. If you are the oncoming student, acknowledge to your team the prior student's help. This sharing will provide the best care to the patients, make both students look good, and help your likely overworked intern. (If you think you are tired in medical school, just wait until you get to residency!)

2. Student to resident

Students should try to help their residents and fellows whenever possible. In the course of my career, I was definitely the most stressed and fatigued during the residency portion. I know this to be true for most surgical residencies, and I know many medical residents have to work hard, too. Teaching the medical students on the team takes time and energy from the residents, so make sure the resident knows you appreciate his efforts.

The best way to be helpful is to learn what has to be done and to do it. When you start on a service, you will likely be given a list of duties (obtain morning vitals, get notes ready, gather dressing supplied needed for rounds). Make sure that you do these things! This sounds basic, but I cannot tell you how often they did not get done when we had certain students on our team. If you do not know how to do something, just ask. Do not say you will do something when you know you will not be able to do it, either because you do not know how or you have other things you were told you have to do first. If someone assigns you a task and you do not do it, the person will be mad.

Try not to ask your resident, "What do you want me to do?" This can actually make MORE work for the resident in trying to find a task you can accomplish. Instead, you should try to figure out what needs to be done on your team and which of those things you would be able to do. For example, you could ask, "Would you like me to talk to the physical therapist about our concerns with Ms. Walker?" Or, "Would you like me to remove Mr. Chen's drain?" If it is something where you need help, you could say, "Would you be able to show me how to do Mr. Gregg's dressing change at noon so I can do the 4:00 P.M. change myself?" This shows that you are paying attention to things, demonstrates initiative, and helps the residents. Sometimes if your resident is really busy, he just needs you to be quiet and let him get his work done. Try to be aware of this so you are not pestering him with questions, even if they are offers of assistance.

As with fellow students, try to make your residents look good. If you have learned an important piece of information about a patient, share it with your resident. Don't hide it and then try to "impress" your attending with it later. This may do harm to the patient and will probably make your resident less likely to try to teach or assist you. You probably know a lot more about Yakamoto-Franklin-Obscuro disease than your resident since you spent 4 hours preparing a presentation about it, but don't act superior. Your resident may have listened to you give a practice talk, so you can acknowledge her for that. Residents like knowledgeable medical students, but not cocky ones. In team rotations as opposed to preceptorships, a lot of your evaluation is probably coming from your residents. So even if it is only to get a high score, you want to be on their good sides.

3. Student to attending

As a medical student, I was under the impression that it was most important to impress the attending. However, in a lot of situations, the attendings will have limited interactions with the students. You do want to make sure you make a positive impression on the attending, but it may not really mean much in your performance evaluation. Try to make sure the attending knows you are a part of the team by being available, but do not make a nuisance of yourself by dominating the attending's time. Do spend face time with them whenever possible, but not in an annoying way.

If possible, introduce yourself whenever you meet an attending. Do not interrupt her in the middle of talking to a patient or during a technically challenging portion of a surgery, but tell her who you are as soon as possible. As a resident, I have seen attendings ask, "Who was that person who was just here?" when the student did not introduce himself. Even if you correctly answered all of their questions, they did not know who you were!

Do not overtly try to impress them. You might impress an attending with your knowledge, but generally not by giving him a spontaneous lecture on above-noted Yakamoto-Franklin-Obscuro disease. No one likes to feel ignorant. When the attending talks about going skiing last weekend, do not talk about how you are the junior triple black diamond champion and have been to all the best resorts in Colorado. You MIGHT choose to say, "Oh, I like to ski, too," but even this can be risky. As an attending and a resident, I wanted the student to be focused on learning. If the student could answer all of my anatomy questions and had all of the patients' lab results ready, then it was OK to talk about social things. Otherwise, the student needed to spend more time focusing on the task at hand. Only when you can take out tonsils in your sleep should you be listening to music or talking about your weekend plans while in surgery, and you probably haven't reached this level as a medical student.

Although I said you shouldn't actively try to impress attendings, you DO want to impress them through your behavior and scholarship. Show up on time. This is such a simple thing, but does not always happen. As a medical student, you rarely have an appropriate reason to be late for something. You are usually not the main person in charge of patient care, so you should show up on time — or better yet, early. Be professional. This includes treating colleagues and patients with respect when you talk to them and about them. Make sure you are studying. If you are going to the pediatric asthma clinic the next day, read as much as you can about pediatric asthma leading up to it.

Do take advantage of "roundsmanship." If an attending asks you a somewhat obscure question but you know the answer because you happened to read about it the previous day, answer the question correctly. You should NOT say, "I had never heard about this until last night, but then I found this section about it in my textbook." The attending does not have to know that you got lucky!

Chapter 3: Residents and fellows

You finally have the M.D. or D.O. after your name, but a lot of people still don't think you're a doctor. You are given little respect. You've got a mountain of debt and you only make $12 an hour (at least that's what I calculated for myself intern year). You work really hard, get very little sleep, and always need more time to study. The good news is that you WILL learn a lot — and you will eventually finish your training.

1. Residents to students

Remember, you were once a student. Most students are trying their best, even if they are not being effective. Be nice to them. Hopefully they have read the previous chapter so they know how to help you.

Set clear expectations for the student. If a student doesn't know she is supposed to come in early to collect the vitals and check on any overnight events, she probably isn't going to do it. If the student has not been told what to do, it is unfair for you to get angry with the student when it isn't done. Make sure you tell students when and where to show up, appropriate dress code, and responsibilities. When interviewing a patient together, let the student know who is supposed to be talking. When I am doing the interview, I don't want the student to butt in. If I am letting the student lead the interview, I will try to hold my questions until the end. If a student doesn't know how you are supposed to work together, it will likely be disorganized and frustrating.

Teach your student. As a resident, you sometimes feel like you don't know very much. There is probably still something you can teach your medical student, whether it is where to find dressing supplies, how to perform and interpret the cardiac exam, or the best way to interact with a certain attending. Students are ultimately there to learn, and as the resident, you are usually the person spending the most time with them.

2. Residents to residents

There is a lot of hierarchy even within residency, including interns, junior/mid-level residents, and senior/chief residents. Ultimately, the residents on a service should function together as a team, with roles usually laid out by the attending or chief resident. The team needs to make sure that each person knows his duties so everything gets done. If there are weak members of the team, the person in charge needs to make sure jobs are assigned appropriately so the work gets done. As a mid-level resident on an inpatient service, I was angry when one of my interns did not complete the tasks that I had assigned to him. My chief pointed out that the intern had poor time management and prioritizing skills, so I had set him up to fail by assigning more work than he could handle. Ideally, we want everyone to be a top-caliber performer, but realistically, we need to get everything done. I don't want to have to do more than my fair share of work, but if that is what it takes to provide good patient care and let the team go home before 10 P.M., that is what I need to do.

Another important piece of resident communication is patient sign-out. When most of the team goes home, you need to make sure that the residents still in charge of the patients know the relevant information. We had spreadsheets for each of our services that included each patient's name, medical record number, age, allergies, surgery date, procedure description, hospital summary, and "to-do" list. Other services had similar information in a list created from the EMR. Whenever we were changing shifts, we would go over the list in person or on the phone. The covering resident should have a chance to ask questions to make sure the plan is clear. If sign-out is not good, it is easier for problems to occur. If I forget to tell the night resident to check on Mr. Zeller's INR, his surgery might be delayed the next day.

Many of the other tips for residents seem like common sense, but it can still help to spell them out. One of my surgery chiefs once said to me, "Common sense isn't very common." This often seems true in medicine — not to mention life in general. As residents, treat each other with respect. Everyone is ultimately trying to learn during residency, even more so than in medical school. Try to teach each other what you have already learned. Do not throw other residents "under the bus." If a certain resident has a particular behavior issue that needs to be addressed, do it with that person in private. If the behavior is dangerous and the attending or administration needs to be involved, inform the appropriate person in a confidential manner.

3. Residents to attendings

For me, the way the attendings treated me in residency changed a lot as I progressed through the program. I felt that as an intern rotating through my home ENT service, the majority of attendings didn't know (and seemingly didn't care) who I was. As a PGY-2 and 3, they wanted to test me to see if I could survive, including very long hours and frequent "pimping." As a chief, I was treated as their colleague and felt that they respected my opinions (most of the time). It was definitely a frustrating process, but I ultimately survived.

As a resident, I think it is sometimes hard for us to understand that the attendings would generally not be there if they weren't interested in teaching us. They could probably make a lot more money and work shorter hours outside of an academic environment. Some subspecialties may only be available within an academic setting so a physician may be forced to work with residents to be able to practice in his niche, but I think that is really the minority of academic attendings. I know that this is not going to be your mindset when you have been up all night caring for patients and Dr. Padayar is quizzing you the next day about the pharmacokinetics of the newest diabetes medication, but at least acknowledge the thought every once in a while.

That being said, I think there is a difference between teaching and tormenting. Some attendings have a very derogatory demeanor towards residents, whereas others are more encouraging. You want to prepare as much as possible so you are ready when the next pimping session arrives, but it is nearly impossible to learn everything. If you have not studied or have done something wrong, part of the attending's job is to try to correct that. He may do it in front of your colleagues, which is usually undesirable for you, but may help everyone learn. Unfortunately, medicine has a different culture from many other industries. If a supervisor treated employees the way some attendings treat residents, the supervisor would be fired. However, if you feel like the critique or behavior from an attending is actually becoming abusive, you can always talk to another resident, the program director, or administration. This may not produce the result that you want, but there are at least a few things that are too egregious even for the training environment.

The best way to avoid critique is to do a good job. You need to make sure you are aware of lab results of your patients, knowledgeable about their medical problems, and up to date with any necessary paperwork. You need to work hard — and work smart. If you spend 30 minutes reading an article on the latest innovation in laparoscopic appendectomy instead of talking to the OR control desk and taking the steps to get your acute appendicitis patient down to the OR, your attending will not be happy. You will generally need to study — a LOT — during residency. You learn a lot of important core information in medical school, but I think about 95% of what I use on a daily basis in my practice came from residency. Attendings usually know if you are studying or not — and will sometimes directly ask you about it. Take advantage of roundsmanship when you can, though, just like the medical students.

Try to treat the attendings with respect. They have worked hard to be in their positions, and they are sacrificing some things to teach you. Thank them when they teach you something, and then show the ultimate appreciation by putting it into practice to help your patients. I had the opportunity to work with many different attendings during my training. I definitely preferred some styles and techniques over others, but I generally had to do things the way the attending instructed. Unless something an attending tells you to do is likely to harm a patient or colleague, you generally need to follow his orders.

Chapter 4: Attending physicians

In medical school and residency, we always called the physicians who had completed their residency attendings. Outside of the academic world, it seems like most people just talk about "providers" or "physicians." Since I have never been an academic attending physician, I do not have as much information specific to this section, but I have mentored a couple students since starting my practice. I will use this section to tell attendings what I would have liked from them as a medical student and resident.

1. Attendings to medical students

Try to remember back to your first clinical rotation as a student. Many of us were very excited to finally be seeing patients and working with a team, only to have an attending ignore us, berate us, or talk way over our heads. Depending on the structure of a rotation, you will have varying interactions with a student. In a team setting, the student may be working mostly with the residents. In a preceptorship, you might be 1-on-1 with the student. Whatever the situation, make sure you and the student are getting as much out of your time together as possible. If you are talking about different chemotherapy protocols for Burkitt's lymphoma but your student has never heard of the disease or the drugs, neither of you are really accomplishing anything. Try to assess the student's knowledge level and tailor your instruction to her when able.

Set expectations for the student. This may be verbal or written. If the student does not live up to the expectations, determine if it is a problem with the student or with the expectations. If you tell a student to show up at a certain time, she should do so unless she has a required class during that time that she has mentioned to you. If you expect the student to be able to close an incision with a running subcuticular stitch without any instruction, that may be unreasonable.

2. Attendings to residents

In the US, residency is designed to teach residents what they need to know to be able to go out and practice independently in their specialty. After completing medical school, you have very little of that information under your belt. Through study, working with attendings, and seeing patients, you (hopefully) acquire the necessary information over a 3- to 9-year period.

One of my attendings described the phases of "physicianhood" to me. You start out being "unconsciously incompetent." Basically, you are not aware of the fact that you don't know anything. You then reach "conscious incompetence," where you know that you don't know things. Somewhere along the way, you transition to "unconscious competence," where you can actually do a lot of things well but do not yet know it. Hopefully, you eventually reach "conscious competence," where you know you know and can do things. I like to add a final stage of "conscious humility." In this stage, you know that you have learned a lot, but there is still a lot more to be learned, both by you and the medical field. I don't think this stage usually comes until after you have finished residency.

As an attending, please remember these stages that one has to progress through during residency. You should expect a resident to show improvement, but she will generally not be able to do things as quickly or as proficiently as you. Residents in the first two stages will need more supervision and guidance than those in the later stages. As a resident, I wanted to know that my attending was there if I needed her, but I also needed space to work on more independent decision-making and surgical skills. I most enjoyed working with attendings who were able to achieve that balance.

As a former resident, I ask attendings not to be cruel just because they can. Residents have to do what you tell them to do for the most part, but they will be much less miserable if you treat them with care and respect. As a junior resident, I was often hurt by things attendings would say to me. For example, if you cut through even a small vessel without cauterizing sufficiently, one of our surgeons liked to say, "Doctor, did you not see that blood-containing structure?" When I was a senior resident and saw them saying the same things to a junior resident who was doing a good job overall, I realized that what I had thought was a serious critique was really more of a teasing remark. When you are not sure of your skills and are sleep-deprived, it is often hard to interpret the meaning behind a comment. As a chief, when an attending would say something like this, I would either let the junior know not to worry about it or throw the same sort of thing back at the attending. If you are an attending with this jeering style, please make sure you let the residents know when they are doing a good job in addition to pointing out their mistakes.

Chapter 5: Other providers

Unless you are a PCP in solo practice and you have very healthy patients, you are usually not the only provider caring for an individual patient. This chapter gives tips on communication with other physicians and mid-level providers.

1. Mid-level providers

I have worked with nurse practitioners (NPs) and physician assistants (PAs), as well as mid-level anesthesia providers (CRNAs and AAs). Mid-level providers go through different training pathways than physicians, but many are still very good at their jobs.

As a junior resident, I did not understand how to work with mid-levels as I had never been exposed to them before. The ENT service was all residents and attendings, but some of the other hospital services utilized mid-levels. When calling a hospital ward, I would usually ask to talk to the resident or attending taking care of patient X (as opposed to the nurse). If a PA came on the phone, it was kind of confusing. We need to understand the concept of "equivalent providers." A mid-level may take the role of a resident on a particular service, so we need to interact with him the way we would a resident.

If you have a mid-level on your service, it is helpful to know each person's role. We added a NP to our head and neck cancer service when I was a senior resident, and it was her job to facilitate patient discharges and be the initial contact on the ward for the nurses. This freed the residents to try to get to the OR so we could get surgical experience. At the VA hospital, our PA worked as the surgery scheduler and saw outpatients in the clinic. Relationships between mid-levels and residents sometimes seemed strained, but it was much better when we each knew our responsibilities.

When I was a resident, some mid-levels seemed to resent being told what to do by a resident. I did not see it as any different than telling my junior resident to complete a task since we were all on the same team, but I sometimes got push-back from a mid-level. One option is to phrase things differently. For example, you can ask rather than tell — "Jane, could you please check Mr. Carey's labs at noon?" If appropriate, you can acknowledge that the instruction is coming from an attending. "Mark, Dr. Ang wanted me to have you see that new consult and report back to him."

Be respectful toward mid-levels. They do not have inferior knowledge or skills just because they did not go to medical school. A CRNA who has been in the OR for 10 years will usually provide smoother anesthesia for the surgeon and patient than a PGY-2 anesthesia resident, or even some of the full anesthesiologists who are more used to supervising than being a front-liner. I have seen NPs and PAs referred to as "physician-extenders" in the medical literature, but when I used that term with an administrator, he was offended. He felt that our NP had his own practice and should not be seen as someone who merely helps the physicians. I did not intend the term in that way, but I mention it to you as a cautionary tale.

Since mid-levels go through a different training pathway, try to teach them things that you know. We currently have an NP in our department who runs his own clinic. He refers the surgical patients to the physicians and asks us questions when he is unsure of something. When I see an interesting case or have a little extra time, I will often ask if he is familiar with a certain concept and then share some of the things I have learned. For example, I talked to him a couple weeks ago about how to describe certain types of hoarseness and the pathophysiology behind the different vocal qualities. I also played a voice sample of a patient with a fairly uncommon but distinctive-sounding condition called spasmodic dysphonia. He told me the next week that he ended up seeing a patient with the condition the very next day! People say you don't really know something unless you can teach it, so it is helpful for me to teach when possible. It is clearly beneficial for our NP and his patients, as well.

2. Physicians in your own specialty

If a physician graduated from the same residency program as you in the same year, you probably received about the same training. If not, you may have learned very different things. If you are partners in a practice, you need to make sure you elucidate any important care differences so you know how to counsel their patients when you are covering call for each other. It is nice to standardize some things if possible, as well. For example, you might have a rule in your group that you will only refill emergency medications after hours and instruct patients to call back the next day for all other prescriptions.

ENT is a fairly small specialty, so I know at least by name all of the other ENT physicians in Albuquerque. Although we are in some ways competing with each other, I am grateful that we have generally collegial relationships. I may end up seeing patients who are unhappy with another ENT doctor they have seen, but I'm sure that goes both ways. If I disagree with the way another physician does something, I will keep that to myself unless I feel that it is actually jeopardizing the patient. I will usually give the patient a recommendation as to what I would do and why, but I do not "bad-mouth" other physicians to patients.

3. Physicians in other specialties

Many patients will have physicians from multiple specialties caring for them, both as inpatients and outpatients. These physicians need to communicate to provide the best care for each patient. If you have a shared EMR that everyone can access, placing timely detailed notes is the simplest way. If something is urgent or confusing, try to have a conversation with the appropriate physician. If a hospitalist calls me to request a consult, I usually ask her at that time if she wants me to just leave a note in the chart or to call back, as well, after I have seen the patient.

Whenever you refer a patient to another physician, you should try to make sure that the physician has as much information as possible. Send along your clinical notes, relevant lab results, and operative note. If imaging studies have been performed and you do not know if the physician will have access to them, instruct the patient to take disks of these studies. When a patient is referred to me, I always make sure to send the referring physician my note so he knows the results of my assessment. If the patient sees multiple physicians, I will usually ask if there is anyone else that should get a copy of my note.

Try to respect the knowledge of each type of physician. ED providers and PCPs have sent me patients for "tympanic membrane perforations," but when I examine the patient, I see that it is just scarring of the eardrum. Non-ENT providers do not have the benefit of the same equipment and specific ear training that we get in ENT. On the flip side, they are much better at listening to the heart and interpreting an ECG than I am at this point in my career. It can be confusing for patients to get contradictory information, so I try not to give a diagnosis if I am not sure about something. If a patient is sent to me for headaches but their sinuses are normal, I may refer them on to a neurologist, who I describe to the patient as a "headache specialist." I will not diagnose the patient with migraines even though I might suspect that, since I am not well-versed in the diagnostic criteria. Similarly, if a PCP sends a dizzy patient to me, it makes more sense for the PCP to say "dizziness" rather than "Meniere's disease" unless the patient has really met all of the criteria for that diagnosis.

4. The difficult colleague

Just as we have some "difficult" patients, you will have a hard time working with certain colleagues. If there is an endocrinologist that you don't like but there is another endocrinologist you can refer to instead, do that as a start. Avoidance is not always an option, though. If the problem is that someone is just rude or mean to you but you are forced to work with her, you may have to put aside your feelings so you can care for the patient together. It might be appropriate to talk to her about some of your concerns, but I cannot guarantee any outcomes. In these types of conversations, it is usually most helpful to start by stating the facts and describing your feelings. For example, "When you said you would refer Mr. Edwards to someone else after I expressed my concerns about doing a surgery, I felt frustrated because it seemed like you hadn't heard my rationale." You do not want to accuse the other person of "being a jerk" or call her names. Listen to her side of the story, as well, and see if you can make a plan together to try to work things out for future interactions. I will sometimes ask other colleagues if they have had similar problems with a certain individual, as it can be helpful to know it is not just me. You can always complain to your friends or family as an outlet, but beware of social media and any HIPAA issues.

If you disagree with the way another physician practices, you have to ask yourself if it is just a style issue or if it is actually dangerous to patients. I may think my way of managing hypertension is superior to

Dr. Cole's, but if he is still within the clinical norms, there is not much I can or should do about it. If I know Dr. Cole, I might ask him why he generally chooses beta blockers over ACE-inhibitors, but I cannot make him change his practice.

On the other hand, if a physician is doing something that you think or know is dangerous, you cannot allow it to continue. Depending on the circumstance, you may be able to talk to the colleague first. For example, if you see that your colleague has shown up late to work on multiple occasions and has been very distracted in caring for patients, you can ask what is happening. You may be able to tell him about the employee assistance program to get him needed counseling. In other situations, such as sexual harassment, you may need to go right to the person's supervisor or the authorities.

<u>Chapter 6: Ancillary staff</u>

As if working with all the people above is not confusing enough, you will encounter a lot of other health professionals who care for your joint patients. This includes nurses, various therapists, and care coordinators.

1. Nurses

I was told when I started residency, "Nurses can be your best friends or they can make your life miserable." Nurses are usually the people who have the most direct contact with inpatients and actually deliver most of the care (medications, suctioning, dressing changes, assessing pain, talking with the patient). However, their scope of practice is limited in that they need an order from a physician to do most of their work. If you make a nurse angry, she may wait until midnight to call you for a Benadryl order to help the patient sleep. If you work well with her, she may catch you on afternoon rounds and ask if you can put it in as a PRN so she will not have to call you later. It makes sense to be nice to nurses just because it is the right thing to do, but it can also come back to hurt you if you are not.

In addition to taking good care of your patients on the floor, nurses can help you personally. My first rotation as an intern was the surgical ICU, where we had a high volume of very sick patients. On my first day, I was asked which pressor and what dose to give a patient. The nurse suggested starting norepinephrine at a certain rate. I was very grateful to her because I had no idea of the specifics. I could have found my senior and asked or tried to look it up, but it was extremely helpful to have nurses who knew what to do. Nurses also know what supplies they have on the floor and where they are kept. They can help you get things for bedside procedures, as well as administering needed medications. Pre-op nurses can alert you to the fact that your outpatient surgery patient does not have a ride or any other problems that come up during check-in.

2. Therapists

In ENT alone, I work with physical therapists, occupational therapists, speech/swallow therapists, and voice therapists. I know there are likely even more with other specialties. These individuals do important work with the patients that I am unable to do, either from my lack of knowledge or lack of time. I have not really had problems communicating with the therapists, as it is usually a situation where you place an order and they see the patient. However, it is helpful for you to know how to best utilize their skills.

I may be able to give a patient a list of exercises to help with his condition, but it is usually much more effective to have someone actually take the patient through the exercises and give him as much explanation as needed. Most therapists perform some sort of evaluation when seeing a new patient, and then tailor the intervention to that patient. They will then follow up and add or change exercises as needed.

The "therapy" word in the title of all these professionals is often key. In addition to various physical and mental exercises, these therapists are often very good at listening to patients and addressing their concerns. In a 20-minute office visit with a new patient with dyspnea, I have to take a history of her symptoms, review all of the past medical history, review the pulmonology note and findings, perform an exam, perform laryngoscopy to look at the vocal cords, explain my findings and recommendations, and place orders for any referrals or medications. She may tell me that her breathing problems started when she was going through a stressful divorce, which may lead me to suspect vocal cord dysfunction, but I do not have time to go into the details of how that stress affected her. I also do not have the training to really teach her the coping skills to deal with the physical and emotional ramifications of the event. The voice therapist has the time and training to do most of these things.

3. Care coordinators

Over the past 10 years, I have seen a significant increase in various "care coordinator" positions. Medicine has grown increasingly complex with paperwork, insurances, costly or multi-step treatment, and diversity of healthcare personnel. Patients are also living longer, including some very ill patients. Care coordinators can be very helpful in these situations.

I do not know how care coordinators started, but it seems to me like a combination of social workers and administrative nurses. You may work with either or both of these types of professionals, as well, so I am including them together here. The two main named coordinator positions I have worked with are discharge planners and cancer nurse navigators.

When a patient is discharged, we have to arrange a location (home, SNF, rehab, LTACH, etc), medications, therapies, and follow-up. When this is complex, it definitely helps to have a specialist in this arena. In surgical services, it also frees the residents to get to the OR to learn necessary surgical skills. In working with a discharge planner, you need to tell them when the patient is likely to be ready for discharge, specific discharge needs, and discharge disposition. You need to update him as soon as possible if any of these plans change. Our general rule in residency was to do whatever the discharge planner needed whenever he needed it (scripts, discharge plan in the EMR, signatures on SNF forms). It definitely made our jobs easier.

I have also been fortunate to have a cancer nurse navigator (CNN) at several of my practices. This is a nurse who helps patients and their families work through the complicated maze of cancer care. The CNN helps arrange appointments with radiation oncologists, medical oncologists, surgeons, and therapists. She can help arrange transportation and financial assistance. She can explain why patients have to see the various specialists and be a contact person for both patients and physicians. In even the fairly small city of Albuquerque, we have 3 separate medical systems as well as many independent providers. The CNN helps streamline and organize care to help reduce fragmentation. If you have a CNN, tell her what you need for the patient and keep her informed so she can help you and the patient as much as possible.

Chapter 7: Industry

I generally think of "Industry" as a necessary evil. In case you are not yet aware of the industry term, I am basically talking about drug and device representatives and their companies. We clearly need companies to make medications and medical equipment, but I don't want the individuals selling these things to take up much of my time. The best way to control your interactions with representatives is to make sure that you have boundaries and expectations in place. However, there can be some benefits to your relationship with industry, as well.

1. Access

Many hospital systems have their own rules about when and how industry reps can access the facilities or the physicians. This will often protect you from having people showing up at your office unannounced. If your practice does not have rules, you can make your own and communicate them to your office staff. For example, you can tell them that you will only meet with reps on the third Tuesday of each month from noon to 12:30. Or you can require staff to screen all reps through you and you will tell them when to meet. You can also tell your staff that you will not meet with reps at all unless you request the meeting. I feel that it is very disruptive to have someone "stop by to chat" any time she feels like it, so I definitely use limits for the reps.

You can also choose how to be in contact with the reps. It can all go through your staff, or you can be the main contact person. Personally, I would not recommend giving a rep your cell phone number, but that choice is up to you. I use my work e-mail to contact the few reps that I actually need, but do not give even that out to many reps. Some reps will be very respectful of your time and not barrage you with visits, calls, or e-mails, but others will not. I prefer not to give them the opportunity.

2. Services and gifts

Although I have discussed above the negative side of industry, there are also things to be gained through your relationship with reps. They do have the most up-to-date information about new products. They are usually happy to provide you with research studies and indications. You need to read these things critically, though, as the research is often sponsored by the manufacturer.

In addition to information, they may provide you with complimentary products. Again, many hospital systems have limits on gifts from industry, so make sure you abide by your institution's policies. Some reps will provide free samples of medications, which can be especially helpful for low-income patients. You might be able to try a new device — like a certain stapler or biologic dressing — in the operating room free-of-charge for the first few cases.

Companies will sometimes sponsor meetings or courses that can give you new skills or CME credits. In residency, I went to a cadaver dissection course in Florida sponsored by one of the device manufacturers. One of the laser companies provided a course at our home institution that gave all of the residents certification in laser safety and use. I also went to a plating course in Pittsburgh where I received hands-on instruction in facial fracture repair. As a resident, these were all free services provided to me by various companies. Less of this is available when you are out in practice, but you may still be able to find good experiences.

All of the services above are gifts to some extent. Regulations on gifts from industry have become much stricter, so just make sure you comply with any institutional and ethical guidelines. You also often have to disclose any relationships with industry as potential biases, such as being a paid speaker or having funding for research. If a rep offers to bring lunch for the office so they can tell you about a new medication, I would recommend that you have them coordinate it through your clinical manager or medical staff affairs department to make sure you do not break any rules. Or if you don't want to meet with him, just say no!

Chapter 8: Researchers

My husband is a researcher (non-medical), so I have a definite affinity for the researcher-type. He can sit silently for hours with only his pencil, paper, and brain. He loves to think about the fine details of an esoteric concept that is understandable to only a fraction of a percent of the educated population. When you have a patient who is coding, though, it is difficult to reconcile the two worlds.

My residency included a 4-month research block in the PGY-3 year. Most of us did bench-top research with various PhDs associated with the department. I worked on several projects in hearing research using a mouse model. We still took evening and weekend hospital call during the research block, but our days were generally free for research. We did sometimes get pulled if another resident was on vacation and we needed to fill in in the operating room or if there were too many cases for the regular team to cover. We had a great relationship, but my professor often seemed irritated when clinical responsibilities pulled me away from the lab. I would have preferred to do research over being awake all night dealing with a patient complication, but I did not really have a choice as a resident.

As physicians, we have chosen a field where our primary job is to take care of the patients. Researchers have a different objective — to gain new knowledge. Any time you are starting a project with a researcher, you should make sure you communicate the fact that you might be pulled away by patient care obligations.

You should try to minimize these interruptions as much as possible, but it is unlikely that you can eliminate that risk.

As a PGY-4, I helped one of the anatomy professors teach the advanced head and neck anatomy course. We tried to schedule lectures around my known clinical obligations, but there were a couple times where I was pulled away for emergencies. Other residents tried to help cover, but I was sometimes the only person available. The professor was understanding, but he could not replace my clinical experience when I was not there.

I think we have a lot to gain by working with researchers, so do not let this difference in priorities discourage you. Many are highly intelligent people who are making the discoveries we need to move medicine forward. Just make sure you communicate with each other so everyone has the best possible experience!

SECTION THREE: Communication with Everyone Else

Chapter 1: Yourself

Medical training is hard. You don't sleep enough, you are asked to do a lot of physically and psychologically demanding tasks, and you receive very little appreciation for all of your work. It often felt to me that no one was thinking about me as a person, so I had to make sure I was aware of myself. If you can't do this, you'll probably be pretty miserable, and you won't be able to communicate effectively with anyone else.

1. Be true to yourself.

You were a person before you became a medical student or doctor. You had values, hobbies, and goals. Hopefully your career in medicine will help reinforce some of these things, but you will at times find yourself being pushed in directions you do not like. If you are asked to do something you know is wrong, do not do it. Some of your values and ideas may change during your training, but do not let yourself turn into a person you do not like or respect.

That being said, you do have to be aware of situations so you do not needlessly offend those around you by "being yourself." You may have to suppress some of your personality traits at times, but you can still find ways to express them. I have kind of a goofy sense of humor. As a junior resident, this was generally saved for home and friends. As a senior resident and now attending, I can use it at work with certain colleagues. I would sometimes tell my junior residents, "Slow your roll," to communicate in a way that would lighten their day. I sometimes sing or dance a little in the OR. Once I know people and have earned their respect, I feel I can be more myself. I stay professional with patients, but can sometimes use a joke or two. I was performing a myringotomy in the office (making a small cut on the ear drum to release trapped fluid). Right before I started, my patient told me she watched a video of it on YouTube. I told her that that was how I had learned to do it and we both got a good laugh. Although it might get suppressed, try not to lose your sense of humor during your training.

In addition to who you are, pay attention to what you want. Is your goal to take care of the most complex patients, be involved in clinical research, work in a remote area with the underserved, focus on "bread and butter" cases, have a predictable work schedule, live in a certain area of the country, or make the most money you can? There is no right or wrong answer — you just have to make sure that you are working toward your particular goal. You may choose to work really hard right out of residency to make a lot of money so you can then have more freedom to choose other paths. Being involved with training the next generation of doctors may be most important to you. Your medical school or training program may try to push you in one direction, but you have to make sure you identify your individual goals so you can tailor your practice to meet those goals. Even if your medical school is one of the top 5 research institutions in the world, you may not want to incorporate research into your practice. That is OK. You have to be comfortable with what you choose to do.

Listen to your inner voice. If something doesn't feel right, take a step back and analyze the situation. You will almost never regret not doing surgery, but you sometimes regret doing it. If you did not have a strong indication for a surgery but you do it anyways and have a complication, it can have serious consequences. If you get a bad gut feeling about a patient and operate on her, she is basically yours forever. If it is medically appropriate for you to do the surgery, make sure you are very clear about possible complications and expected outcomes. If you are concerned, do not be afraid to refer to a colleague for a second opinion. Do not do anything you think is dangerous or may cause harm, even if someone above you in the hierarchy tells you to do so.

2. Find time for yourself.

This is hard when you collapse as soon as you get home. The "time for yourself" as a resident may be 5 minutes here and there, but you still need to do it. One of my favorite times of day in residency was when I was taking a shower. I knew I could not answer my pager for those 5-10 minutes, which gave me a little sanity break when things were crazy.

When you do have time off, make sure you enjoy it. My husband and I would often go on walks to the nearby lakes on free evenings when we happened to get nice weather (which could be hard in Cleveland). I always tried to have something fun planned when I actually had a vacation. It did not have to be an expensive trip, but we would go camping or at least spend time with friends. I never used vacation to write a paper or do other work-related tasks, although I know some of my colleagues did. I knew I needed that time away from work. You will probably use some of your time off to catch up on sleep, but make sure you do something you like, as well.

A lot of people find relaxation in exercise. It has never worked for me — I just feel more tired! — but I feel I should mention it here. It is well known that there are physical and psychological benefits to exercise. It is often a good way to focus on yourself, too, and exclude outside distractions.

Chapter 2: Family and friends

Unless your family and friends are in medicine, they will not understand what you are going through in your training. You often have more freedom when you get into practice, but you will most likely still have some call or holiday obligations.

1. Significant other

I married my wonderful, supportive husband right before starting medical school, so I was lucky. I did see some married couples divorce during medical school and residency, due at least in part to the strain the job places on relationships. It is usually hard for non-medical people to understand the time and energy you must put into your training and the near-total lack of control you sometimes have over your schedule. When you're woken up in the middle of the night by page after page, it might be waking up your spouse, as well. I know I'm not a very pleasant person when I'm constantly tired, either, so it takes a caring partner to put up with that. I tried very hard not to take out my frustrations on him, but he definitely heard a lot of complaining and crying.

Although you constantly have to work on a relationship, I have to think that it is even harder to start a new relationship when you are spending so much time at work. If you are not already in an established relationship, ask yourself what you want. Do you want to devote time and energy to finding that special someone? Or do you want to avoid anything serious at this point? I would recommend that you try to set expectations for anyone you date — e.g., "I may not be able to call you during the week since I will be working from 6 A.M. to 8 P.M. each day and then have to prepare for my grand rounds presentation," or, "I don't have a free weekend again until next month, but let's try to get together then."

You need to make sure that your significant other knows he or she is important to you even if you do not get to spend as much time together as you would like. Ever since we got married, I have told my husband that I love him at least several times each day. I ask him about his day. He asks about my day, although he sometimes gets more than he bargained for. You don't want to inundate your spouse with complaints, but he or she is there to support you "for better or for worse." Like I said before, I don't think I could have made it through medical school and residency without the support of my husband. Even though my job as a full physician now is better, I still look forward to coming home to him every day.

2. Family

My parents are great people, but I don't think they ever understood how little control I had over my schedule in residency. I would often hear something like, "We are getting together next weekend for Easter. Can you come?" If I planned a month or two in advance, I might be able to get a free weekend, but it was nearly impossible to do things on short notice. Our program flat out did not allow us to take vacation during certain times, such as the month of July or the Christmas holiday. There were required weekend and evening events. Things are easier now, but I still do not have as much free time as I would like.

I think the best ways to cope with scheduling challenges are to try to plan things as far in advance as possible and to explain to your family early on that you may not always be available. I tried to call my parents each weekend, but I did not get to see them very often during medical school or residency. You often have geographic limitations in medical school, and a request but no actual choice in residency with the match system. When you choose where to practice, you can decide how geographic proximity to family affects your choice. My husband and I wanted to move out west, but we made sure we were in a city that had an airport so we could get back to family when needed.

I do not have any children, but I know some people who had children in medical school and residency. Multiple people have told me that you can always find an excuse to put off having children until later, but that you should just go ahead and start a family when you want to. I have seen people make it work, but I don't think it was something I would have been able to do in medical school or residency. I feel that if I choose to have children, I need to make sure I have enough time to spend with them. I would not want to miss out on their childhood or have someone else raise my children. Since I am not a parent, I cannot fairly critique most parenting choices, but these are my opinions. Don't rush into children without thinking, but don't let anything hold you back if that is what you really want. If you have a stay-at-home spouse or available family nearby, that definitely helps.

You also have to make sure that you can continue your clinical duties while caring for your children, especially if you have them during your training. When I was a chief resident, one of our PGY3s had a baby. After that, he was constantly 10 minutes late to rounds due to dropping his child off at day care. He liked the day care because it saved him a lot of money over having a private nanny, but it was not acceptable for him to always be late to work. He eventually had to find a different solution, even though it cost more. If you are going to continue to work while you have children, you have to make sure your work does not suffer, either.

3. Friends

Since I moved to new places for medical school and residency, most of my friends were going through training with me. It was definitely easier to maintain this type of friendship since we all recognized the various challenges of the training process. Even with that, though, some of my resident friends would say, "You kind of disappeared for a few months there when you were on the head and neck surgery rotation." It was sad we did not get to spend as much time together as we wanted, but we understood.

It is generally harder for non-medical friends. As with family and significant others, make sure they know what to expect. If you won't be able to see them for a while, try to let them know ahead of time. You don't want them to think you don't call them because you don't care — you're just really busy! It's good to try to have some non-medical friends to help remind you that there is a world outside of medicine. It's nice to have occasional conversations about music and sports instead of diabetes and diverticula.

Chapter 3: Social media

I did not grow up with today's technology, so I am not an active user of most forms of social media. One of my medical school friends recently posted a link on Facebook identifying us as the 'Oregon Trail Generation.' I was in middle school when my family got a home computer, complete with dial-up modem. I had one of the bulky car phones in high school since my mom worried when I drove to the community college. I joined Facebook during my residency but never got into the newer, 'cooler' apps.

In a profession like medicine, you always have to remember to be careful with social media. Although you can retract posts, people can repost things almost immediately. There was recently a local nurse who posted on Facebook that she was having a slow night at work and wished someone would code so she would have something to do. She was fired immediately, and I highly doubt she will be able to keep her nursing license. I'm sure she did not mean what she said, but once things are out there on social media, you cannot really get rid of them. Some employers will look at you on social media as part of their hiring decision. Be careful in who you share social media with, as you probably do not want your boss to see pictures of you drunk with your friends. I use Facebook to post pictures of trips and check on what my friends are doing, but I make sure not to post anything controversial or patient-related. HIPAA applies to social media, as well, so I strongly advise you not to mix work with social media.

Conclusion

I have tried to make this an easy-to-read book as I know we are usually quite busy in our medical practice and training. Even if it is a quick read, I hope it makes you think about how you are interacting with your patients, other professionals, and the world around you. If I had known when I started what I know now, I think there would have been less pain along the way. I am not perfect by any stretch of the imagination, so I hope you can learn from some of my mistakes rather than making them all yourself. We have chosen a professional where communication is critical. I hope you are able to take some of the keys from this book and use them throughout your career.

Good luck!

www.ingramcontent.com/pod-product-compliance
Lightning Source LLC
Chambersburg PA
CBHW051340170526
45166CB00002B/888